MW00574685

Ketogenic Bread Cookbook for Beginners

Thomas Slow

Table of Contents

Introduction

Congratulations on purchasing *Keto Bread* and thank you for doing so. Inspiration for a special way of eating is what sent me on the keto journey. I have heard many good things about the plan as you too will soon discover. If you're new to the keto diet plan, let's discover a bit of the history of how the diet has traveled through time.

During the Paleogenic period, humans were known to hunt for their protein and gather their vegetables, fruits, nuts, and seeds to survive. Because this method isn't ideal in today's society; you don't have to search for food each day. That was the way people lived centuries ago which made the body develop a mechanism to survive during times when food was scarce.

Whenever a person encountered satiation where they consumed more calories than they burned, the unused calories would be converted into fat fuels and stored for emergency starvation times. This mechanism was useful in times where nutrient resources were scarce and required a lot more energy to locate.

However, in modern times, food is not the only natural to come by, but most meals that are affordable are packed full of unnecessary calories. Your body will continue to create these fat stores, even though the times of hunting and gathering are behind us. These facts were taken into consideration when the ketogenic diet was developed.

The only way to lose fat is to trick the body into burning it. If you specifically consume meals high in fats and very low-lacking in carbohydrates; your body will believe that the only fuel available is fat. It will then enter what is known as ketosis; the process whereby the liver releases more ketones. Thus, ketones form as a result of burning fats for fuels.

Starvation mode is known when the body is calorie deficient and lacking in the nutrients it needs. Many people have forced his/her bodies into starvation mode in a desperate attempt to lose weight. However, what few people realize is that the weight loss while in starvation mode is usually muscle tissue. The body holds onto its emergency fat stores until the last possible moment. A ketosis is a form of starvation mode that takes this fat away. You won't be depriving your body of calories or nutrients. You will be starving your body of carbohydrates and sugars.

During the era of the 1920s and 1930s, the ketogenic diet was prevalent for its role in epilepsy therapy treatments. The diet plan provided another method other than the uncharacteristic techniques of fasting which were victorious in the treatment plan. During the 1940s, the process was abandoned because of new therapies for seizures. However, approximately 20 to 30% of the epileptic cases failed to reach control of epileptic seizures. With that failure, the keto diet was reintroduced as a management technique.

The Charlie Foundation was founded by the family of Charlie Abraham in 1994 after his recovery from seizures and other health issues he suffered daily. Charlie—as a youngster—was placed on the diet and continued to use it for five years. As of 2016, he is still functioning successfully without the seizure episodes and is furthering his education as a college student.

The Charlie Foundation appointed a panel of dietitians and neurologists to form an agreement in the form of a statement in 2006. It was written as an approval of the diet and stated which cases its use would be considered. It is noted that the plan is especially recommended for children. The plan continues to improve as time passes and more research is completed.

Chapter 3: Keto Bread Recipes

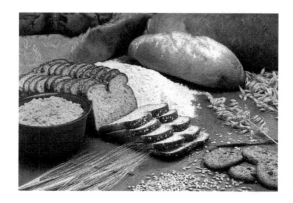

Gluten-Free Cranberry Bread

Yields Provided: 12 Servings

Macro Counts For Each Serving:

- **Fat Content**: 15 g
- **Total Net Carbs**: 4.7 g
- **Protein**: 6.4 g
- **Calories**: 179

List of Ingredients:

- Almond flour (2 cups)
- Powdered erythritol or Swerve (.5 cup)
- Steviva stevia powder (.5 tsp.)
- Bak. powder (1.5 tsp.)
- Bak. soda (.5 tsp.)
- Salt (1 tsp.)
- Unsalted butter melted or coconut oil (4 tbsp.)
- Eggs at room temperature (4 large)
- Coconut milk (.5 cup)
- Cranberries (12 oz. bag)
- _Optional_: Blackstrap molasses (1 tsp.)
- Also Needed: 9x5-inch loaf pan

Preparation Technique:

1. Program the oven temperature to reach 350° Fahrenheit. Lightly grease the baking pan before you start baking.

2. Sift the flour, baking powder, baking soda, erythritol or stevia, salt.

3. In a container, combine the eggs, butter, molasses, and coconut milk.

4. Combine it all until well combined.

5. Fold in the rinsed cranberries, and add to the pan.

6. Bake about 1.25 hours. Watch closely when you approach the 1-hour marker since oven temperatures vary.

7. Arrange the pan on a rack to cool (15 min.) before removing from the pan.

Keto 90-Second French Toast

Yields Provided: 2 Servings

Macro Counts For Each Serving:

- **Fat Content**: 30 g
- **Total Net Carbs**: 4 g
- **Protein**: 12 g
- **Calories**: 352

List of Ingredients:

- Coconut flour (1 tbsp.)
- Melted butter (1.25 tbsp.)
- Egg (1)
- Cream cheese (1 tsp.)
- Bak. powder (.25 tsp.)
- Nutmeg (1 pinch)
- Cinnamon (.25 tsp.)

List of Ingredients - The Toast:

- Egg (1)
- Heavy whipping cream (.25 cup)
- Lakanto Monkfruit Powdered Sugar (.25 tsp.)
- Optional: Sugar-Free Maple Syrup

Preparation Technique:

- Melt butter in a glass bowl (6-inch).
- Work in the remainder of the fixings, whisking until combined.
- Cook for 1.5 minutes in the microwave.
- Transfer to the countertop to cool for a minute or two. Cut the bread in half.
- In a flat dish; whisk one egg and 1/4 cup of the heavy whipping cream.
- Soak both sides of bread in egg/whipping cream mixture.
- Heat one tablespoon of butter in a skillet and fry each side until crispy.
- Sprinkle 1/4 teaspoon of the Swerve Confectioners' Sugar and serve with sugar-free syrup. Berries are also delicious.

Keto 90-Second Bread

Yields Provided: 4 Servings

Macro Counts For Each Serving:

- **Fat Content**: 9 g
- **Total Net Carbs**: 2 g
- **Protein**: 3 g
- **Calories**: 90

List of Ingredients:

- Coconut flour (1 tbsp.)
- Almond flour (.25 cup)
- Coconut oil (1 tbsp.)
- Bak. powder (.25 tsp.)
- Egg (1)

Preparation Technique:

- Combine all of the fixings in a microwave-safe cup or ramekin. Mix well.
- Microwave for 90 seconds.
- Carefully transfer the bread from the microwave. Cool for one to two minutes.
- Cut in half and serve.

Low-Carb Zucchini Walnut Bread

Yields Provided: 8 Servings

Macro Counts For Each Serving:

- **Fat Content**: 36 g
- **Total Net Carbs**: 6 g
- **Protein**: 10 g
- **Calories**: 397

List of Ingredients:

- Truvia or your favorite sweetener (.5 cup)
- Eggs (3)
- Ghee or Oil (.5 cup)
- Almond flour (1.5 cups)
- Bak. powder (1 tsp.)
- Coconut flour (.5 cup)
- Bak. soda (1 tsp.)
- Nutmeg (.25 tsp.)
- Cinnamon (.5 tsp.)
- Unsweetened almond milk (.5 cup)
- Chopped walnuts (1 cup)
- Shredded zucchini (2 cups)
- Also Needed: 6-cup bundt pan

Preparation Technique:

- Set the oven at 350° Fahrenheit.

- Grease the pan and set aside.
- Toss the eggs, sweetener, and oil into the stand mixer mixing bowl. Use the paddle attachment to beat for 2 to 3 minutes until well incorporated.
- Add the coconut and almond flour, baking powder, nutmeg, baking soda, cinnamon, and almond milk. Continue mixing for another two to three minutes.
- Stir in the shredded zucchini and chopped walnuts and arrange in the greased pan.
- Bake for 30 minutes. Cool slightly to serve.

Macadamia Bread

Yields Provided: 16 Servings

Macro Counts For Each Serving:

- **Fat Content**: 22 g
- **Total Net Carbs**: 5 g
- **Protein**: 5 g
- **Calories**: 227

List of Ingredients:

- Macadamia nuts (2 cups)
- Eggs (4)
- Almond flour (.25 cup)
- Ground flaxseed (2 tbsp.)
- Softened ghee (.25 cup)
- Softened coconut butter (.5 cup)
- Sea salt (1 tsp.)
- Bak. powder (.5 tsp.)
- Apple cider vinegar (2 tbsp.)
- _Also Needed_: 8 x 4 loaf pan

Preparation Technique:

1. Warm up the oven to 350° Fahrenheit.
2. Lightly grease the pan with ghee.

3. Process the nuts using the food processor until they are a fine flour.
4. Crack and add the eggs with the motor running until the mixture is creamy.
5. Fold in the flaxseed, almond flour, coconut butter, ghee, vinegar, sea salt, and baking powder. Continue processing until well combined.
6. Scoop in the oiled bread pan.
7. Bake for 35 to 40 minutes. Cool the bread before slicing to serve or store.

Pork Rind Bread

Yields Provided: 12 Servings

Macro Counts For Each Serving:

- **Fat Content:** 13 g
- **Total Net Carbs:** 1.9 g
- **Protein:** 9 g
- **Calories:** 166

List of Ingredients:

- Cream cheese (8 oz.)
- Grated mozzarella cheese (2 cups)
- Large eggs (3)
- Grated parmesan cheese (.25 cup)
- Crushed pork rinds (1 cup)
- Baking powder (1 tbsp.)
- Herbs and spices (as desired)
- _Also Needed_: Loaf pan - 5 by 9-inch

Preparation Technique:

1. Set the oven temperature to reach 375° Fahrenheit.
2. Prepare a baking tin with the paper.
3. Place both types of cheese into a safe dish. Microwave using the high-power setting for one minute. Stir and microwave for another minute.

4. Fold in the egg with the parmesan, baking powder, and pork rinds. Stir until all ingredients have been incorporated. Spread onto the pan.
5. Bake for 15 to 20 minutes. When ready, add the pan to a cooling rack for about 15 minutes.

Pumpkin Bread

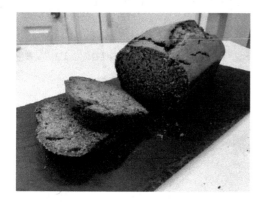

Yields Provided: 12 Servings

Macro Counts For Each Serving:

- **Fat Content**: 18 g
- **Total Net Carbs**: 4 g
- **Protein**: 8 g
- **Calories**: 215

List of Ingredients:

- Blanched almond flour (2 cups)
- Coconut flour (.5 cup)
- Erythritol (.75 cup)
- Pumpkin pie spice (2 tsp.)
- Sea salt (.25 tsp.)
- Gluten-free bak. powder (2 tsp.)
- Pumpkin puree (.75 cup)
- Eggs (4 large - lightly beaten)

- Butter (measured solid, then melted; can use ghee or coconut oil (.33 cup)
- Pumpkin seeds (.25 cup)
- *Also Needed*: Loaf pan 9 by 5-inches

Preparation Technique:

1. Warm the oven to reach 350° Fahrenheit
2. Prepare the pan with parchment baking paper. Leave some of the bag hanging over the edges for easy removal later.
3. Sift or whisk the coconut flour, erythritol, almond flour, pumpkin pie spice, sea salt, and baking powder.
4. Fold in the pumpkin puree, eggs, and melted butter. Mix well.
5. Empty the batter into the lined pan. Sprinkle the top with pumpkin seeds and press them lightly into the surface.
6. Bake for 50 minutes to one hour.
7. Cool completely before removing from the pan and slicing.

Savory Stuffed Bread

Yields Provided: 10 Servings

Macro Counts For Each Serving:

- **Fat Content**: 20 g
- **Total Net Carbs**: 2 g
- **Protein**: 6 g
- **Calories**: 202

List of Ingredients:

- Baking powder (1.5 tsp.)
- Parsley seasoning (2 tbsp.)
- Sage (1 tsp.)
- Rosemary (1 tsp.)
- Medium eggs (8)
- Cream cheese (1 cup)
- Butter (.5 cup)
- Almond flour (2.5 cups)
- Coconut flour (.25 cup)

Preparation Technique:

1. Warm the oven to reach 350° Fahrenheit. Grease a loaf pan.

2. Cream/smash the butter and cream cheese. Fold in the seasonings (parsley, sage, and rosemary).

3. Whisk and break in the egg to form the batter until it's smooth.
4. Combine the almond and coconut flour with the baking powder.
5. Mix all of the fixings until well incorporated.
6. Scoop into the loaf pan.
7. Set the timer and bake for 50 minutes. Serve and enjoy.

Sesame Seed Bread

Yields Provided: 6 Servings

Macro Counts For Each Serving:

- **Fat Content**: 13 g
- **Total Net Carbs**: 1 g
- **Protein**: 7 g
- **Calories**: 100

List of Ingredients:

- Boiling water (1 cup)
- Almond flour (1.25 cups)
- Bak. powder (2 tsp.)
- Sesame seeds (2 tbsp.)
- Psyllium husk powder (5 tbsp.)
- Sea salt (.25 tsp.)
- Apple cider vinegar (2 tsp.)
- Egg whites (3)

Preparation Technique:

1. Set the oven temperature to reach 350° Fahrenheit.
2. Oils the baking sheet. Put water in a saucepan to boil.
3. Mix the sea salt, baking powder, almond flour, sesame seeds, and psyllium powder.

4. Stir in the hot water, vinegar, and egg whites. Use a hand mixer (less than 1 min.) to combine. Place the bread on the prepared pan.

5. Bake for one hour on the lowest oven rack. Serve and enjoy any time.

Yields Provided: 4 Servings

Macro Counts For Each Serving:

- **Fat Content**: 8.2 g
- **Total Net Carbs**: 1.9 g
- **Protein**: 3.5 g
- **Calories**: 107

List of Ingredients:

- Chia seeds (.25 cup)
- Sunflower seeds (.5 cup)
- Pumpkin seeds (.5 cup)
- Coconut flour (.25 cup)
- Psyllium husks (1 cup)
- Bak. powder (1 tsp.)
- *Optional*: Salt (.25 tsp.)
- Melted butter (.5 stick)
- Eggs (2 medium)
- Warm water (1 cup)

Preparation Technique:

1. Toss all of the dry fixings into the mixing container. Whisk well.
2. Melt the butter. Whisk in the eggs until almost mixed.

3. Pour in warm water and stir until all the ingredients are fully incorporated.

4. Place in a loaf tin and bake at 350° Fahrenheit for 35 to 45 minutes.

Delicious Buns

Garlic & Basil Buns

Yields Provided: 8 Servings

Macro Counts For Each Serving:

- **Fat Content**: 15 g
- **Total Net Carbs**: 1.4 g
- **Protein**: 9.6 g
- **Calories**: 186

List of Ingredients:

- Water (.75 cup)
- Butter (6 tbsp.)
- Salt (1 pinch)
- Chopped fresh basil (1 cup)
- Crushed garlic cloves (6)
- Eggs (4)
- Almond flour (.75 cup)
- Grated parmesan (5.5 oz)

Preparation Technique:

1. Warm up the oven to 400° Fahrenheit.
2. Cover a baking tin with a layer of parchment paper.
3. Boil the water and add the salt and butter.

4. Take the pan away from the heat and add the flour. Combine well, and break in the eggs.

5. Fold in the garlic, basil, and lastly, the parmesan.

6. Once it's creamy, add the dough on the prepared pan one spoonful at a time while shaping into buns.

7. Bake for 20 minutes and enjoy. Cool before storing.

Poppy Seed Buns

Yields Provided: 12 Servings

Macro Counts For Each Serving:

- **Fat Content**: 11.5 g
- **Total Net Carbs**: 6.2 g
- **Protein**: 10.6 g
- **Calories**: 162

List of Ingredients:

- Eggs (6 whites & 2 whole)
- Salt (.5 tsp.)
- Psyllium husk powder (.33 cup)
- Coconut flour (.5 cup)
- Almond flour (2 cups)
- Boiling water (2 cups)
- Cream of tartar (1.5 tsp.)
- Garlic powder (2 tsp.)

- Baking soda (1.3 tsp.)
- Poppy seeds (2 tbsp.)

Preparation Technique:

1. Warm up the oven to reach 350° Fahrenheit.
2. Combine all of the dry fixings.
3. In another dish, add all of the eggs and whisk. Pour in the boiling water and continue stirring.
4. Combine everything and stir until mixed well.
5. Spoon into the pan. Bake for 20 to 25 minutes.

Spring Onion Buns

Yields Provided: 6 Servings

Macro Counts For Each Serving:

- **Fat Content:** 6.7 g
- **Total Net Carbs:** 1.1 g
- **Protein:** 4.2 g
- **Calories:** 81

List of Ingredients:

- Separated eggs (3)
- Stevia (1 tsp.)
- Cream cheese (3.5 oz.)
- Baking powder (.5 tsp.)
- Salt (1 pinch)

List of Ingredients - For the Filling:

- Chopped hard-boiled egg (1)
- Diced spring onions (2 sprigs)

Preparation Technique:

1. Warm up the oven to 300° Fahrenheit.
2. Spritz the muffin cups with some oil.
3. Combine the egg yolks, stevia, cream cheese, salt, and baking powder.

4. Whisk the egg whites in another cup.

5. Combine the fixings with a spatula, and add the dough to the muffin cups.

6. Combine the filling components and add them to the cups. It is important to fill the cups only half full to allow room for the rest of the fillings.

7. Pour additional dough into the cup. Bake for 30 minutes.

8. Cool slightly and serve.

Tasty Biscuits & Focaccia

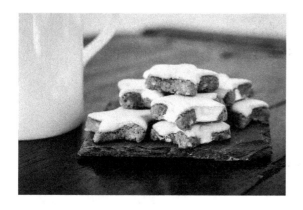

Keto Sausage Biscuits

Yields Provided: 6 Servings

Macro Counts For Each Serving:

- **Fat Content**: 20 g
- **Total Net Carbs**: 2 g
- **Protein**: 12 g
- **Calories**: 250

List of Ingredients:

- Cream cheese (2 oz.)
- Mozzarella (2 cups - shredded)
- Eggs (2)
- Almond flour (1 cup)
- Salt & pepper (1 pinch of each)
- Colby jack cheese/another favorite (2 oz.)
- Pre-cooked breakfast sausage patties (6)

Preparation Technique:

1. Warm the oven to reach 400° Fahrenheit. Prepare a muffin tin with a spritz of cooking oil.
2. Thinly slice the Colby jack into chunks or squares into a microwave-safe container, adding the mozzarella and cream cheese. Cook at 30-second intervals until softened and melted.

3. Whisk the egg and almond flour. Combine with the cheese mixture.
4. Place on a layer of plastic wrap, and pop into the fridge until firm.
5. Slice into six 3-inch balls. Flatten the balls, place the sausage on the dough, sliced cheese, and wrap the dough around.
6. Arrange in the muffin tin.
7. Bake until set or for 10 to 15 minutes. Top with additional cheese as desired.

Low-Carb "Red Lobster" Mimic Biscuits

Yields Provided: 10 Servings
Macro Counts For Each Serving:
- **Fat Content**: 22.4 g
- **Total Net Carbs**: 1.8 g
- **Protein**: 6.2 g
- **Calories**: 230

List of Ingredients:
- Almond flour (2 cups)
- Baking powder (2 tsp.)
- Garlic & Onion powder (.5 tsp. each)
- Kosher salt (.5 tsp.)

- Freshly cracked pepper (1 pinch)
- Green onions (.25 cup - finely sliced)
- Eggs (2 beaten)
- Melted butter (.5 cup)
- Cheddar cheese shredded (.5 cup)

Preparation Technique:

1. Set the oven to 350° Fahrenheit. Prepare a cookie sheet with a layer of parchment paper.
2. Sift or whisk the almond flour. Add the baking powder, salt, couple cracks of pepper, onion and garlic powder, green onions, and mix well.
3. Whisk the eggs and melted oil with the rest of the fixings. Lastly, add the shredded cheese and stir well.
4. Fill a ¼ cup measuring cup about ¾ full of dough. Form the dough into a ball and place it on the paper. Repeat with remaining dough, making sure they are not too close to each other.
5. Bake until golden brown (22 min.). Remove and cool for 15 minutes before serving.

Rosemary & Olive Focaccia Bread

Yields Provided: 10 Servings

Macro Counts For Each Serving:

- **Fat Content**: 26 g
- **Total Net Carbs**: 3.5 g
- **Protein**: 8 g
- **Calories**: 284

List of Ingredients:

- Unchilled cream cheese (4 oz.)
- Unchilled salted butter (4 oz.)
- Baking powder (1 tsp.)
- Xanthan gum (.25 tsp.)
- Large eggs (4)
- Almond flour (1.50 cups)
- Garlic powder (.5 tsp.)
- Rosemary (3 sprigs)
- Kalamata olives (16)
- Also Needed: 8 by 12-inch baking pan

Preparation Technique:

1. Set the oven temperature to reach 375° Fahrenheit.

2. Cover a baking pan with a sheet of parchment baking paper.
3. Place the butter and cream cheese into a mixing container. Whip (high speed) using a hand mixer until fluffy.
4. Fold in the eggs one at a time and beat well.
5. Add the baking powder, flour, xanthan gum, and garlic powder. Stir well with a mixing spoon and scoop the dough onto the baking tin.
6. Top using olives, and rosemary.
7. Bake for 19-25 minutes, or when the focaccia springs back when touched.
8. Enjoy warm or cool to slice as a delicious sandwich at any time.

Sour Cream Biscuits

Yields Provided: 10 Servings

Macro Counts For Each Serving:

- **Fat Content**: 16 g
- **Total Net Carbs**: 3.2 g
- **Protein**: 6 g
- **Calories**: 190

List of Ingredients:

- Coconut flour (.33 cup)
- Almond flour (1.5 cups)
- Hemp seed (2 tbsp.)
- Swerve (1 tsp.)
- Bak. soda (.5 tsp.)
- Salt (.5 tsp.)
- Bak. powder (2 tsp.)
- Sour cream (.5 cup)
- Egg (1)
- Melted butter (2 tbsp.)
- Cream (2 tbsp.)
- Water (2 tbsp. or more as needed)

Preparation Technique:

1. Set the oven at 450° Fahrenheit.

2. If you're using an iron skillet, let it get hot also.

3. Whisk the almond flour, salt, hemp seed, baking soda, baking powder, coconut flour, and sweetener.

4. Whisk the egg, sour cream, melted butter, cream, and water.

5. Combine all of the fixings using gentle strokes. Set aside for now.

6. Toss the butter or bacon grease into the hot skillet. Add the biscuits to the skillet and return the skillet to the oven.

7. Bake for 12 to 15 minutes.

8. Transfer to the countertop. Cool before serving.

9. Serve warm with butter or your favorite low-carb toppings.

Yields Provided: 1 Serving

Macro Counts For Each Serving:

- **Fat Content**: 32 g
- **Total Net Carbs**: 4.5 g
- **Protein**: 15 g
- **Calories**: 390

List of Ingredients:

- Butter (1 tbsp.)
- Coconut flour (2 tbsp.)
- Egg (1 large)
- Heavy whipping cream (1 tbsp.)
- Water (2 tbsp.)
- Garlic powder (.125 tsp.)
- Baking powder (.25 tsp.)
- Onion powder (.125 tsp.)
- Cheddar cheese (.25 cup)
- Dried parsley (.125 tsp.)
- Pink Himalayan Salt (.125 tsp.)
- Black pepper (.125 tsp.)

Preparation Technique:

1. Melt butter in a coffee cup in the microwave for 20 seconds.
2. Mix in the baking powder, coconut flour, and seasonings using a fork.
3. Stir in the egg, cheese, water, and heavy cream.
4. Microwave for three minutes. Carefully, remove the cup and cool for two minutes.
5. Slice and enjoy.

Chapter 4: Keto Muffins

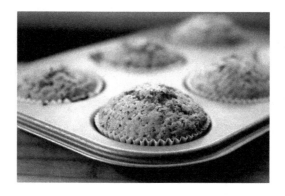

Coffee Cake Muffins

Yields Provided: 12 Servings

Macro Counts For Each Serving:

- **Fat Content**: 18 g
- **Total Net Carbs**: 5 g
- **Protein**: 7 g
- **Calories**: 224

List of Ingredients - For the Batter:

- Unchilled butter (2 tbsp.)
- Unchilled cream cheese (2 oz.)
- Stevia or favorite sweetener (.33 cup)
- Eggs (4)
- Vanilla (2 tsp.)
- Unsweetened vanilla almond milk (.5 cup)
- Almond flour (1 cup)
- Bak. powder (1 tsp.)
- Coconut flour (.5 cup)
- Salt (.25 tsp.)

List of Ingredients - For the Topping:

- Almond flour (1 cup)
- Coconut flour (2 tbsp.)
- Softened butter (.25 cup)

- Cinnamon (1 tsp.)
- Stevia/your choice (.25 cup)
- *Optional*: Molasses (.5 tsp.)
- *Also Needed*: Standard muffin tin & Parchment baking paper

Preparation Technique:

1. Soften the butter and cream cheese for about 30 minutes on the countertop before preparing the recipe.
2. Warm the oven to reach 350° Fahrenheit.
3. Prepare the tin with a spritz of cooking oil spray.
4. Combine all the batter fixings in a food processor. Mix thoroughly and pour into the muffin tin.
5. Combine the topping fixings in the processor. Pulse until crumbs form. Sprinkle on top of the batter.
6. Bake 22-25 min until golden.
7. *Note:* If the crumb topping starts to get too dark cover with foil for the last 5 minutes.

Cranberry Orange Muffins

Yields Provided: 14 Servings

Macro Counts For Each Serving:
- **Fat Content**: 11.2 g
- **Total Net Carbs**: 9.3 g
- **Protein**: 6.1 g
- **Calories**: 197

List of Ingredients:
- Coconut flour (1.25 cups)
- Eggs (8)
- Powdered vanilla bean (1 tsp.)
- Bak. soda (.5 tsp.)
- Unsalted butter or ghee - melted (.5 cup + extra for greasing)
- Fresh cranberries (1 cup - lightly crushed)
- Birch xylitol (1 cup + 1 tbsp.)
- Orange zest (1 tbsp.)
- Salt (.5 tsp.)

Preparation Technique:
1. Set the oven to 355° Fahrenheit.
2. Whisk the coconut flour, orange zest, baking soda, vanilla powder, xylitol, and salt.

3. Add eggs and butter into the flour mixture. Mix then add the cranberries.

4. Prepare a muffin tin with butter or use muffin liners.

5. Divide batter evenly amongst the muffin tin forms.

6. Bake for 27 to 35 minutes. Serve warm.

"Double The Choc" Moist & Sweet Muffins

Yields Provided: 12 Servings

Macro Counts For Each Serving:

- **Fat Content**: 26 g
- **Total Net Carbs**: 4 g
- **Protein**: 7 g
- **Calories**: 300

List of Ingredients:

- Almond flour (1 cup)
- Erythritol (.5 cup)
- Eggs (3)
- Heavy cream (.66 cup)
- Unsweetened cocoa powder (.5 cup)
- Bak. powder (1.5 tsp.)
- Melted butter - unsalted (3 oz.)
- Vanilla extract (1 tsp.)
- Sugar-free chocolate chips (.5 cup)
- *Also Needed:* 12-count muffin tin

Preparation Technique:

1. Heat the oven to 350° Fahrenheit.
2. Combine the erythritol, almond flour, baking powder, and cocoa powder.

3. Mix in vanilla extract, heavy cream, and eggs. Melt, then add the butter and chocolate chips. Stir.

4. Spoon the mixture into holes of a standard muffin tray that has been lined with cupcake papers.

5. Bake 22 minutes.

Feta & Spinach Muffins

Yields Provided: 6 Servings

Macro Counts For Each Serving:

- **Fat Content**: 16 g
- **Total Net Carbs**: 2 g
- **Protein**: 14 g
- **Calories**: 209

List of Ingredients:

- Eggs (6)
- Bacon (3 slices - cooked)
- Raw spinach (2 cups)
- Crumbled feta cheese (1 cup)
- Cheddar cheese (.5 cup)
- Black pepper & salt (as desired)

Preparation Technique:

1. Warm the oven in advance to reach 350° Fahrenheit.
2. Rinse the spinach under cold water. Drain, and toss into a microwave-safe container. Cook on high for one minute. Set aside for a few minutes.
3. In another mixing container, whisk the eggs until frothy.
4. Fold in grated cheddar cheese, feta cheese, and bacon pieces.

5. Once the spinach is cooled enough, add to the bowl and mix until combined. Divide into the six muffin cups.
6. Bake for 32-35 minutes until muffins are firm.

Flaxseed Muffins

Yields Provided: 12 Servings

Macro Counts For Each Serving:

- **Fat Content**: 20 g
- **Total Net Carbs**: 2 g
- **Protein**: 6 g
- **Calories**: 220

List of Ingredients:

- Ground golden flaxseed or buy flax meal already ground (1 cup)
- Eggs (4)
- Avocado oil (.5 cup)
- Granulated sweetener - Lakanto maple sugar erythritol (.5 cup)
- Lemon juice (1 tsp.)
- Cinnamon (2 tsp.)
- Bak. soda (.5 tsp)
- Coconut flour (.25 cup)
- Salt (1 pinch)
- Vanilla extract (2 tsp.)
- _Optional_: Chopped walnuts (1 cup)

Preparation Technique:

1. Warm the oven to reach 325° Fahrenheit. Prepare the muffin tin with paper liners.
2. If starting with whole golden flaxseed, grind it in a coffee grinder, then measure one cup.
3. Mix the fixings in the order they are listed using an electric mixer. Add in walnuts *last* after using a mixer.
4. Bake for 20 to 22 minutes. Serve when ready after slightly cooling.

Gingerbread Muffins

Yields Provided: 5 Servings

Macro Counts For Each Serving:

- **Fat Content**: 13 g
- **Total Net Carbs**: 2 g
- **Protein**: 4 g
- **Calories**: 167

List of Ingredients:

- Non-dairy milk or water (.75 cup)
- Granulated sweetener - your preference (.25 cup)
- Vanilla extract (1 tsp.)
- Coconut flour (.5 cup)
- Ground flax seeds (.5 cup)
- Coconut oil (2 tbsp.)
- Freshly grated ginger (1.5 tsp.)
- Allspice (.25 tsp.)
- Cinnamon (1.5 tsp.)
- Ground cloves (.25 tsp.)
- Nutmeg (.25 tsp.)
- _Also Needed_: Standard-size muffin pan - a minimum of 5-count

Preparation Technique:

1. Warm up the oven to 370° Fahrenheit. Line the pan with baking paper.
2. Combine the flax seeds, oil, milk, and vanilla.
3. Whisk well and wait five minutes for the seeds to rest.
4. In another mixing container, whisk the remainder of the fixings until thickened.
5. Empty the batter into the pan.
6. Bake until the tops are firm to the touch (30-35 min.).
7. Remove and place on the countertop to cool in the pan for at least 15 minutes.
8. Once cool, the muffins should easily pop out of the pan.
9. Store in the fridge until ready to enjoy.

Keto Strawberry Muffins

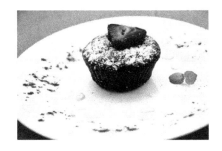

Yields Provided: 12 Servings

Macro Counts For Each Serving:

- **Fat Content**: 11.3 g
- **Total Net Carbs**: 4.5 g
- **Protein**: 6 g
- **Calories**: 211

List of Ingredients:

- Unchilled eggs (3 large)
- Sugar-free crystal sweetener - Monk fruit/erythritol/xylitol (.5 cup)
- Unsweetened vanilla almond milk (.33 cup)
- Melted coconut oil (.33 cup)
- Baking powder (2 tsp.)
- Diced strawberries fresh or thawed (1 cup - 6 oz.)
- Almond flour (2.5 cups)
- 12-count muffin tin

Preparation Technique:

1. Warm the oven to 345° Fahrenheit.
2. Cover the muffin tin with parchment baking paper or grease with an oil spray if preferred. Set aside.
3. Whisk together eggs, sugar-free sweetener of your choice, almond milk, and melted coconut oil.
4. Stir in baking powder and almond flour, 1/2 cup at a time, stirring between to gently incorporate the flour to avoid lumps.
5. Stir in the diced strawberry, with frozen strawberries make sure to defrost them before, eliminate any juice to avoid the muffin batter to get too moist.
6. Transfer the muffin batter evenly into 12 muffin cases.
7. Bake for 22 to 24 min.
8. Cool for 10 minutes then gently remove from pan and cook for at least 30 minutes.

Lemon Poppyseed Muffins

Yields Provided: 12 Servings

Macro Counts For Each Serving:

- **Fat Content**: 13 g
- **Total Net Carbs**: 1 g
- **Protein**: 4 g
- **Calories**: 141

List of Ingredients:

- Eggs (3)
- Full-fat ricotta cheese (.25 cup)
- Coconut oil (.25 cup)
- Poppy seeds (2 tbsp.)
- True lemon packets (4)
- Heavy whipping cream (.25 cup)
- Lemon extract (1 tsp.)
- Almond flour (1 cup)
- Swerve or alternative sweetener (.33 cup)
- Baking powder (1 tsp.)

Preparation Technique:

1. Heat the oven in advance to 350° Fahrenheit.
2. Prepare a 12-count muffin tin with silicone cupcake liners.

3. Combine all of the fixings until smooth. Scrape the batter into the cups.

4. Bake for 38 minutes. Insert a knife or toothpick in the middle of the muffin to check for doneness.

5. Chill for several minutes before taking them from the liners.

1-Minute Keto Muffins

Yields Provided: 1 Serving

Macro Counts For Each Serving:

- **Fat Content:** 6 g
- **Total Net Carbs:** 3 g
- **Protein:** 7 g
- **Calories:** 112

List of Ingredients:

- Egg (1)
- Coconut flour (2 tsp.) or slightly more depending on the brand
- Salt (1 pinch)
- Bak. soda (1 pinch)
- Coconut oil/butter (as needed)

Preparation Technique:

1. Lightly grease the mug with butter/oil.
2. Mix all of the fixings together with a fork to ensure it is lump-free
3. Cook the muffin in the microwave using high for 50 seconds to 1 minute. Cut in half and serve.
4. *Option 2*: Bake for 12 minutes in an oven at 400° Fahrenheit.

5. You can also toast or fry as a side option.

Pumpkin Muffins With Cranberries & Pecans

Yields Provided: 12 Servings

Macro Counts For Each Serving:

- **Fat Content:** 21 g
- **Total Net Carbs:** 5 g
- **Protein:** 5 g
- **Calories:** 238

List of Ingredients:

- Coconut flour (.5 cup)
- Almond flour (1.5 cups)
- Erythritol (.5 cup)
- Salt (.25 tsp.)
- Cinnamon (1 tsp.)
- Canned pumpkin puree (1 cup)
- Bak. powder (3 tsp.)
- Ground ginger (.5 tsp.)
- Eggs (2)
- Melted coconut oil (.5 cup)
- Sugar-free dried cranberries (.5 cup)
- Chopped pecans (.5 cup)
- _Also Needed:_ 12-count muffin tin

Preparation Technique:

1. Prepare the cups and set the oven at 400° Fahrenheit.
2. Mix both types of flour with the sweetener, baking powder, ginger, cinnamon, and salt.
3. Stir in pumpkin, coconut oil, eggs, cranberries, and pecans.
4. Empty into the muffin cups.
5. Bake for 22 to 25 minutes.
6. Cool completely before removing from muffin cups because early removal could cause them to crumble.

3-Way Breakfast Egg Muffins

Yields Provided: 12 Servings

Macro Counts For Each Serving:

- **Fat Content**: 5 g
- **Total Net Carbs**: 1 g
- **Protein**: 6 g
- **Calories**: 82

List of Ingredients- The Base:

- Large eggs (12)
- Finely chopped onion - any color (2 tbsp.)
- Black pepper & salt (as desired)
- Also Needed: 12-cup capacity muffin tin

List of Ingredients - Bacon Cheddar:

- Chopped - cooked bacon (.25 cup)
- Shredded cheddar cheese (.25 cup)

List of Ingredients - Garlic - Mushroom & Pepper:

- Red bell pepper - diced (.25 cup)
- Sliced brown mushrooms (.25 cup)
- Fresh chopped parsley (1 tbsp.)
- Minced garlic (.33 tsp.) or Garlic powder (.25 tsp.)

List of Ingredients - Tomato - Spinach & Mozzarella:

- Grape or cherry tomatoes (8 - halved)
- Fresh spinach - roughly chopped (.25 cup)
- Shredded mozzarella cheese (.25 cup)

Preparation Technique:

1. Warm the oven to 350° Fahrenheit. Spritz the muffin tin with a portion of cooking oil spray.
2. Whisk the eggs, salt, pepper, and onions.
3. Add the egg mixture halfway up into each tin.
4. Divide the three topping combinations into four muffin cups.
5. Bake for 20 minutes.
6. Cool and Serve.

Chapter 5: Keto Cookies

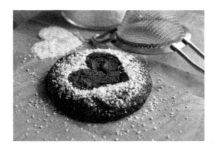

Flourless Chewy Keto Chocolate Cookies

Yields Provided: 15 Servings

Macro Counts For Each Serving:

- **Fat Content**: 15.7 g
- **Total Net Carbs**: 11.3 g
- **Protein**: 5 g
- **Calories**: 173

List of Ingredients:

- Almond butter (1.5 cups)
- Eggs (2)
- Low-calorie natural sweetener - Swerve (.5 cup)
- sifted - unsweetened cocoa powder (.33 cup)
- Sugar-free vanilla extract (1 tsp.)
- Salt (1 pinch)

Preparation Technique:

1. Set the oven to reach 350 ° Fahrenheit. Cover a baking tin with a sheet of parchment baking paper.

2. Blend the eggs, almond butter, salt, cocoa powder, sweetener, and vanilla extract into the bowl of a food processor; pulse until the dough forms.

3. Roll into one-inch balls. Arrange on the cookie sheet, pressing with a fork into a crisscross pattern.

4. Bake about 12 minutes.

5. Cool on the baking sheet for one minute before removing to a cooling rack.

Flourless Keto Cashew Butter Cookies

Yields Provided: 12 Servings

Macro Counts For Each Serving:

- **Fat Content**: 9 g
- **Total Net Carbs**: 2 g
- **Protein**: 5 g
- **Calories**: 103

List of Ingredients:

- Cashew butter (1 cup)
- Granulated sweetener of choice (.75 cup)
- Ground chia seeds (3-4 tbsp.) Can replace with 1 large egg
- Optional: Chocolate chips of choice (1-2 tbsp.)

Preparation Technique:

1. Warm the oven to 350° Fahrenheit. Prepare a cookie sheet with a layer of baking paper.
2. Combine all of the fixings, except for the chocolate chips. Mix. If the cookie batter is too thin, add an extra tablespoon of ground chia seeds. Fold in your chocolate chips.
3. Form 12 small balls of dough and place them on the lined tray. Press each ball in a cookie shape and bake for 10 to

12 minutes, or until just cooked on top and golden edges. Remove from the oven and cool on the tray.

4. Note: Start with 3 tbsp. of ground chia seeds. Only add the extra one if the batter is too thin.

Keto Chocolate Chip Cookies

Yields Provided: 18 Servings

Macro Counts For Each Serving:
- **Fat Content**: 9 g
- **Total Net Carbs**: 1 g
- **Protein**: 2 g
- **Calories**: 96

List of Ingredients:
- Eggs (2 large)
- Pure vanilla extract - alcohol-free (2 tsp.)
- Melted butter (1 stick - .5 cup)
- Heavy cream (2 tbsp.)
- Almond flour (2.75 cups)
- Kosher salt (.25 tsp.)
- Swerve (.5 cup or to taste)
- Dark chocolate chips (.75 cup)

Preparation Technique:
1. Heat the oven to reach 350° Fahrenheit. Prepare the pan with a spritz of cooking oil spray as needed.
2. Whisk the egg with the heavy cream, vanilla, almond flour, butter, salt, and swerve. Fold in the chocolate chips.
3. Form the mixture into one-inch balls.

4. Arrange the cookies about three inches apart onto the cookie sheets.

5. Bake until browned to your liking (17 to 19 min.).

Shortbread Cookies

Yields Provided: 24 Servings

Macro Counts For Each Serving:

- **Protein**: 1 g
- **Fat Content**: 5 g
- **Total Net Carbs**: 1 g
- **Calories**: 59

List of Ingredients:

- Almond flour (1.5 cups)
- Xanthan gum (.5 tsp.)
- Kosher salt (.25 tsp.)
- Unchilled butter (6 tbsp.)
- Powdered erythritol (6 tbsp.)
- Vanilla extract (.5 tsp.)
- *Optional For the Coating*: Melted dark chocolate & Flaky sea salt

Preparation Technique:

1. Sift the almond flour into a dry skillet. Toast using medium heat until golden (3 to 6 min.). Transfer from the pan, whisk in the salt, and xanthan gum. Set aside for now to cool.

2. Cream the butter in a mixing container using an electric mixer (2 to 3 min.).

3. Toss in the vanilla extract and sweetener.

4. With your mixer, slowly add half of the almond flour mixture, stirring until just combined. Add in with the rest of the mixture.

5. Wrap the dough in a cling-type film and store in the fridge for at least an hour.

6. Warm the oven to 350° Fahrenheit.

7. Roll out the dough between parchment paper layers and either simply slices with a knife. Arrange the shaped cookies on a cookie sheet. Place in the freezer for about 15 minutes to firm before baking.

8. Bake using these times; (15 to 18 min. for the larger ones) or (10 to 13 min. for the small ones).

9. Cool the pan because they will crumble when warm.

Tart & Sweet Raspberry Cookies

Yields Provided: 10 Servings

Macro Counts For Each Serving:

- **Fat Content**: 8 g
- **Total Net Carbs**: 5 g
- **Protein**: 3 g
- **Calories**: 132

List of Ingredients:

- Almond flour (1.25 cups)
- Coconut flour (.25 cup)
- Baking powder (1 tsp.)
- Erythritol (.5 cup)
- Raspberries - chopped small (4 oz.)
- Medium egg (1)
- Ghee (1 tbsp.)
- Vanilla extract (1 tsp.

Preparation Technique:

1. Warm the oven to 355° Fahrenheit.
2. Combine the baking powder, coconut flour, almond flour, and sweetener in a bowl. Tip in the chopped raspberries and mix well to combine. Set aside.

3. Whisk the egg and vanilla together. As long as the ghee *isn't* piping hot, drizzle it *slowly* into the egg, whisking continuously until well combined.
4. Pour all of the fixings together and mix.
5. Divide the dough into ten portions. Compress into a ball using your hands, and flatten. Arrange on a parchment paper-lined tray.
6. Bake for 10 minutes, rotating the tray halfway through.
7. Remove and cool completely before enjoying

Vanilla Cheesecake Fat Bomb Snacks

Yields Provided: 18 Servings

Macro Counts For Each Serving:

- **Fat Content**: 9 g
- **Total Net Carbs**: 1 g
- **Protein**: 1 g
- **Calories**: 88

List of Ingredients:

- Cream cheese (9 oz. softened)
- Vanilla extract (2 tsp.)
- Erythritol (2 oz.)
- Heavy cream (1 cup)

Preparation Technique:

1. Soften the cream cheese, and toss with the erythritol and vanilla into a kitchen stand mixer, or mix with a hand mixer using the low speed for two minutes.
2. Add half of the heavy cream and blend for an additional two minutes.
3. Let the bowl sit for three or four minutes.
4. Pour in the rest of the heavy cream and blend using the medium speed setting for three minutes to prepare firm peaks.

5. Fill the mini cupcake liners.

6. Store in the refrigerator for a minimum of one hour before it's time to serve.

Chapter 6: Keto Bagels

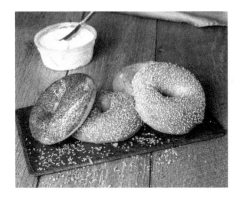

French Toast Bagel

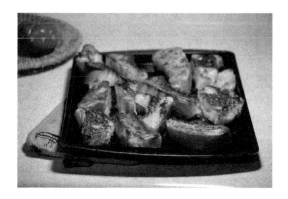

Yields Provided: 6 Servings

Macro Counts For Each Serving:

- **Fat Content**: 16 g
- **Total Net Carbs**: 3 g
- **Protein**: 8 g
- **Calories**: 207

List of Ingredients:

- Eggs (6)
- Cinnamon (1 tbsp.)
- Maple extract (1 tsp.)
- Sugar-free vanilla extract (2 tsp.)
- Sifted coconut flour (.5 cup)
- *Optional:* Xanthan gum or guar gum (.5 tsp.)
- Baking powder (.5 tsp.)

- Stevia glycerite (5-10 drops) or Swerve sweetener (1 to 1.5 tbsp.)
- Melted butter (.33 cup)
- Salt (.5 tsp.)

Preparation Technique:

1. Set the oven temperature at 400° Fahrenheit. Lightly grease the pan.
2. Blend the eggs with the cinnamon, vanilla extract, maple extract, stevia, salt, and butter.
3. Whisk the coconut flour, baking powder, and xanthan gum.
4. Combine everything and spoon into the pan. Bake for 13/15 minutes.
5. Cool thoroughly and store in the refrigerator.

Mozzarella Dough Bagels

Yields Provided: 6 Servings

Macro Counts For Each Serving:

- **Fat Content**: 16.8 g
- **Total Net Carbs**: 2.4 g
- **Protein**: 16.8 g
- **Calories**: 203

List of Ingredients:

- Mozzarella cheese (1.75 cups)
- Salt (1 pinch)
- Almond meal (.75 cup)
- Baking powder (1 tsp.)
- Full-fat cream cheese (2 tbsp.)
- Egg (1 medium)

Preparation Technique:

1. Combine the shredded mozzarella cheese with the cream cheese and almond meal in the mixing bowl. Cook for one minute.
2. Stir the mixture and continue using the high-temperature setting for another 30 seconds.
3. Whisk the egg, baking powder, salt, and any other flavorings.

4. Portion the dough into six segments. Roll into balls and then into cylinder shapes.
5. Fold the ends together to form the bagels. Be sure to secure the ends of the bagels, so they do not become separated during the cooking process.
6. Arrange the bagels on the baking pan and sprinkle with s few of the sesame seeds.
7. Bake at 425° Fahrenheit until golden brown (about 15 min.).

Pizza Bagels

Yields Provided: 6 Servings

Macro Counts For Each Serving:

- **Fat Content**: 35 g
- **Total Net Carbs**: 6 g
- **Protein**: 28 g
- **Calories**: 449

List of Ingredients:

- Baking powder (1 tbsp.)
- Almond flour (2 cups)
- Italian seasoning (1 tsp.)
- Onion powder (1 tsp)
- Large eggs (2 whisked)
- Shredded mozzarella cheese - low moisture (3 cups)
- Cream cheese (3 tbsp.)
- Garlic powder (1 tsp.)
- Low-carb pizza sauce (.25 cup)
- Chopped pepperoni slices (2.5 oz.)
- Dried oregano (1 tsp.)
- Shredded parmesan cheese (2 tbsp.)

Preparation Technique:

1. Set the oven temperature to reach 425° Fahrenheit. Cover a sheet with a layer of baking paper.
2. Sift to combine the almond flour, garlic powder, baking powder, dried Italian seasoning, and onion powder.
3. In a container, combine the mozzarella and the cream cheese. Cook for 1.5 minutes. Remove from microwave and stir to combine. Continue heating at 30-second increments as needed.
4. In a bowl, add the almond flour and the eggs, mix well.
5. Once everything is well combined, mix in the pepperoni to the dough. Little by little, add and mix in the sauce. The dough will be fairly soft.
6. Divide the dough into 6 portions, rolling into a ball.
7. Make a hole in the center and create the bagel shape.
8. Add on the top oregano and parmesan
9. Bake on the middle rack until golden brown or for 12 to 14 minutes.

Yields Provided: 4 Servings

Macro Counts For Each Serving:

- **Fat Content**: 23 g
- **Total Net Carbs**: 4.5 g
- **Protein**: 13 g
- **Calories**: 285

List of Ingredients:

- Salt (.25 tsp.)
- Psyllium husk powder (3 tbsp.)
- Almond flour (1.5 cups)
- Baking soda (.75 tsp.)
- Xanthan gum (.75 tsp.)
- Whole egg (1)
- Egg whites (3)
- Warm water (.5 cup)
- Rosemary (1 tbsp. - chopped)
- Avocado oil

Preparation Technique:

1. Warm the oven at 350° Fahrenheit.
2. Whisk the xanthan gum, baking soda, almond flour, and salt in a container.

3. In another dish, whisk the eggs and warm water. Stir in the psyllium husk.

4. Add the liquid fixings to dry ingredients.

5. Spritz a bagel mold with avocado oil.

6. Press the dough into the mold. Sprinkle rosemary on top.

7. Bake for 45 minutes. Remove and cool for 15 minutes before slicing.

Savory & Sweet Keto Bagels

Yields Provided: 4 Servings

Macro Counts For Each Serving:

- **Fat Content**: 24.6 g
- **Total Net Carbs**: 4 g
- **Protein**: 16.9 g
- **Calories**: 308

List of Ingredients:

- Shredded mozzarella cheese (1.5 cups)
- Almond flour (1 cup)
- Bak. powder (1.5 tsp.)
- Xanthan gum (.25 tsp.)
- Salt (.25 tsp.)
- Egg (1)
- _Optional_:
- Softened butter (3 tbsp.)
- Sukrin Gold brown sugar substitute (3 tbsp.)
- Cinnamon (1 tbsp.)

Preparation Technique:

1. Warm the oven in advance to reach 400° Fahrenheit.
2. Prepare a baking tin using a layer of parchment baking paper.

3. Toss the mozzarella into a dish and microwave using 20-second intervals, until stretchy and melted.
4. Fold in the flour, xanthan gum, and baking powder. Mix well until combined and add the egg to prepare the dough.
5. Arrange the dough onto a sheet of parchment paper and knead into a ball.
6. Slice into four segments and make the 'o' shape for the bagel. Pinch the ends together.
7. Bake until the tops are golden or about 15 minutes.
8. Cool for five to ten minutes before slicing.

Sesame & Poppy Seed Bagels

Yields Provided: 6 Servings

Macro Counts For Each Serving:

- **Fat Content**: 29 g
- **Total Net Carbs**: 5 g
- **Protein**: 20 g
- **Calories**: 350

List of Ingredients:

- Sesame cheese (8 tsp.)
- Poppy seeds (8 tsp.)
- Shredded mozzarella cheese (2.5 cups)
- Baking powder (1 tsp.)
- Almond flour (1.5 cups)
- Large eggs (2)

Preparation Technique:

1. Warm the oven temperature in advance to reach 400° Fahrenheit.
2. Prepare a sheet with a layer of paper. Combine the almond flour and baking powder.
3. Melt the mozzarella and cream cheese in a microwave-safe dish for one minute.
4. Stir and cook one additional minute.

5. Whisk the eggs and add the cheese mixture. Stir and combine with the rest of the fixings. Once the dough is formed, break it apart into 6 pieces.
6. Stretch the dough and join the ends to form the bagels. Arrange on the sheet.
7. Add the seed combination and bake for 15 minutes.

Vegan Keto Everything Bagels

Yields Provided: 6 Servings

Macro Counts For Each Serving:

- **Fat Content**: 25 g
- **Total Net Carbs**: 1 g
- **Protein**: 7 g
- **Calories**: 302

List of Ingredients:

- Melted coconut oil (2 tbsp.)
- Baking powder (1 tsp.)
- Ground golden flaxseed (.5 cup)
- Psyllium husk powder (.25 cup)
- Salt (1 pinch)
- Natural unsweetened, unsalted almond butter (.5 cup)

List of Ingredients - Everything Seasoning:

- Sesame seeds (1 tsp.)
- Garlic flakes (1 tsp.)
- Salt (.25 tsp.)
- Vegan cream cheese - for serving (6 tbsp.)
- Onion flakes (1 tsp.)
- Poppy seeds (1 tsp)

Preparation Technique:

1. Set the oven at 375° Fahrenheit.

2. Grease six sections of a doughnut pan with 1 tbsp. of coconut oil.

3. Stir in the psyllium husk powder, ground flaxseed, baking powder, and salt in a mixing container. Slowly whisk the almond butter with 1 cup warm water until smooth and combined. Add the flaxseed mixture to the almond butter mixture. Stir with a spoon or spatula. Continue to mix until a moldable dough forms. Divide the dough into six portions.

4. Prepare the seasoning. Mix the garlic flakes, poppy seeds, onion flakes, sesame seeds, and sea salt.

5. Press the dough portions into the greased molds. The easiest way to do this is to roll each portion into a long log first, then press it into a mold.

6. Brush the bagel tops with the remaining 1 tbsp. coconut oil. Sprinkle evenly with the seasoning mixture.

7. Bake until golden brown, about 40 minutes.

8. Cool in the pan for 10 minutes before moving to a wire rack to cool completely.

9. Serve each bagel with 1 tbsp. vegan cream cheese.

Chapter 7: Keto Pizza

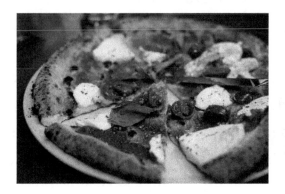

Keto Pepperoni Pizza

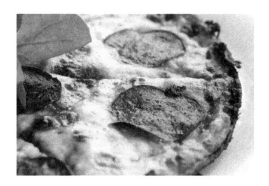

Yields Provided: 6 Servings

Macro Counts For Each Serving:
- **Fat Content**: 27 g
- **Total Net Carbs**: 3.2 g
- **Protein**: 18.2 g
- **Calories**: 335

List of Ingredients - The Base:
- Mozzarella cheese (2 cups/8 oz.)
- Almond flour (.75 cup)
- Psyllium husk powder (1 tbsp.)
- Cream cheese (3 tbsp./1.5 oz.)
- Large egg (1)
- Italian seasoning (1 tbsp.)
- Pepper & Salt (.5 tsp. each)

List of Ingredients - Toppings:

- Mozzarella cheese (1 cup/4 oz.)
- Rao's Tomato Sauce (.5 cup)
- Pepperoni (16 slices)
- *Optional*: Oregano

Preparation Technique:

1. Warm the oven to 400° Fahrenheit.
2. Microwave the mozzarella cheese until completely melted. Add all other base fixings (omit the olive oil) and mix well.
3. Knead the dough into a ball, and spread it out into a circle.
4. Bake the crust for 8 min. Take out from the oven, flip, and bake for two to four additional minutes.
5. Toss the crust with toppings of your choice and bake for another three to five minutes.
6. Let cool slightly before slicing to serve.

Keto Pizza With A Low-Carb Broccoli Pizza Crust

Yields Provided: 4Servings

Macro Counts For Each Serving:

- **Fat Content**: g
- **Total Net Carbs**: g
- **Protein**: g
- **Calories**: 115

List of Ingredients:

- Broccoli rice (two 12 oz. bags) frozen-thawed or fresh (3 cups)
- Large egg (1)
- Garlic powder (.5 tsp.)
- Freshly grated parmesan cheese (.66 cup)
- Optional: Super-fine blanched almond flour, optional but helps to give the crust a crispier texture (2 tbsp.)
- Dried oregano (1 tsp.) optional
- Dried basil (.5 tsp.) optional

List of Ingredients - Topping Options:

- Grated mozzarella (.33 cup)
- Sugar-free marinara sauce (Rao's) or passata sauce (.25 cup)
- Pepperoni (6-8 slices)
- Sliced mushrooms (.25 cup)

- Fresh basil or spinach (3-4 leaves)
- Chopped olives (2-3)

Preparation Technique:

1. Warm the oven in advance to reach 425° Fahrenheit.
2. Arrange the frozen broccoli rice in a microwavable dish and cook using high for three to five minutes. Or, place it in the oven for 10 minutes, rotating the pan and cool for about ten minutes.
3. Combine the prepared broccoli flour, egg, mozzarella, and optional seasonings. Knead well to form the dough.
4. Cover the baking sheet with a layer of parchment baking paper. Add the dough and roll out using a rolling pin to reach about .25 to .5-inch thickness.
5. Make a raised edge and bake for 15 minutes.
6. Remove and add the sauce and desired toppings.
7. Top it off using the mozzarella and bake until the cheese has melted. Slice and serve while piping hot.

Keto Pizza Margherita

Yields Provided: 6 Servings

Macro Counts For Each Serving:

- **Fat Content:** 17 g
- **Total Net Carbs:** 4 g
- **Protein:** 15g
- **Calories:** 237

List of Ingredients - The Fathead Dough:

- Part-skim shredded mozzarella cheese (1.5 cups)
- Almond flour (.75 cup)
- Salt (.5 tsp.)
- Cream cheese (2 tbsp.)
- Egg (1)
- Garlic powder (.5 tsp.)
- Dried oregano (rosemary, thyme, etc. (.5 tsp.)
- Pepper (.25 tsp.)

List of Ingredients - Keto Pizza Margherita:

- Tomato sauce (.25-.33 cup)
- Fresh mozzarella cut into 4 slices (4 oz.)
- Fresh basil leaves (4+)
- *Optional:* Grated parmesan cheese for garnish
- *Optional:* Sprinkle of dried oregano or other seasonings, for garnish

Preparation Technique:

1. Set the oven to 400° Fahrenheit.

2. Add and melt the shredded mozzarella cheese and cream cheese in a non-stick skillet using the medium heat setting, stirring until melted.

3. Transfer to the countertop to rest for 30 seconds.

4. Stir in almond flour, egg, garlic powder, dried seasonings, salt, and pepper; continue to stir until thoroughly combined.

5. Transfer the dough to a parchment paper-lined surface.

6. Add another piece of parchment paper over the dough. Take a rolling pin and place over the top parchment paper; start rolling into a circle until the dough is thin and spread out to about nine inches.

7. If you do not have a rolling pin, wet the palms of your hands with cooking spray and press out the dough into a thin round.

8. Slide the dough onto a sheet leaving the bottom paper attached.

9. Use a fork and dot the dough before adding it into the oven for 10 minutes.

10. If you see any bubbles forming on top of the pizza crust, remove the pie from the oven, poke down with a fork, and continue to bake.

11. When the crust is finished cooking, let stand for a minute.

12. Spread a thin layer of tomato sauce over the pizza crust and add mozzarella.
13. Bake for 7/8 minutes.
14. Remove from the oven, top with fresh basil leaves, sprinkle with parmesan cheese, and oregano to serve.
15. *Note:* To prevent a 'scrambled egg' effect, let the cheese cool for a bit before stirring in the egg.

Mini Keto Pizza With A Crispy Crust

Yields Provided: 1 Serving

Macro Counts For Each Serving:

- **Fat Content:** 26.4 g
- **Total Net Carbs:** 3.5 g
- **Protein:** 15 g
- **Calories:** 325

List of Ingredients - The Bread:

- Coconut flour (1 tbsp.)
- Melted butter (1.25 tbsp.)
- Egg white (1)
- Softened cream cheese (1 tsp.)
- Baking powder (.25 tsp.)
- Grated mozzarella (1 tbsp.)

List of Ingredients - The Pizza:

- Marinara sauce - ex. Rao's (1 tbsp.)
- Mozzarella cheese (.33 cup)
- Favorite toppings
- Italian seasoning to your liking

Preparation Technique:

1. Melt butter in a glass bowl. Toss in and mix the rest of the fixings.
2. Cook in the microwave for 1.5 min. Cool for a minute or two.
3. Heat 1 tbsp. of butter in an oven-proof skillet. Prepare on each side until crisp.
4. Prepare the pizza. Heat the oven to 400° Fahrenheit.
5. Add 1 tbsp. of sauce to the top of the bread and .33 cup of mozzarella cheese. Add the desired toppings. Sprinkle with Italian seasoning.
6. Place the skillet onto the top shelf of the oven. Bake until the cheese is melted (5 to 8 min.).

Mozzarella Crust Pizza

Yields Provided: 2 Servings

Macro Counts For Each Serving:

- **Fat Content**: 20 g
- **Total Net Carbs**: 3 g
- **Protein**: 33 g
- **Calories**: 324

List of Ingredients:

- Mozzarella cheese (2 cups)
- Garlic powder (1 tsp.)
- Pizza seasoning - divided (1 tsp. + 1 pinch)
- Tomato sauce (.5 cup)
- Grated parmesan cheese

Preparation Technique:

1. Set the oven temperature to 400°.
2. Prepare a sheet with a sheet of baking paper (_Not foil_).
3. Sprinkle on the cheese, garlic powder, and a pinch of pizza seasoning.
4. Bake until the cheese is melted (12-15 min.). Cool for about three minutes.

5. Empty the sauce over the top with a sprinkle of parmesan cheese and the rest of the pizza seasoning. Bake for one minute. Slice and serve.

Nut-Free Pizza Crust

Yields Provided: 8 Servings

Macro Counts For Each Serving:

- **Fat Content**: 10.4 g
- **Total Net Carbs**: 1.4 g
- **Protein**: 8.5 g
- **Calories**: 131

List of Ingredients:

- Cream cheese (4 oz. - softened)
- Garlic powder (.5 tsp.)
- Large eggs (2)
- Dried Italian seasoning (.5 tsp.)
- Onion powder (.5 tsp.)
- Grated parmesan cheese (.25 cup)
- Shredded mozzarella cheese (1.25 cup)
- *Also Suggested*: 12-inch pizza pan/baking dish

Preparation Technique:

1. Set the oven to reach 375° Fahrenheit.
2. Cover a pan with parchment paper.
3. Using a hand mixer, combine the cream cheese, eggs, and seasoning.

4. Fold in the parmesan and mozzarella cheese. Scoop into the lined pizza pan.
5. Bake for 22 minutes, flipping halfway through the cooking cycle. To flip it without breaking it, top it with a second sheet of parchment paper, and flip.

Sausage Crust Pizza

Yields Provided: 4 Servings

Macro Counts For Each Serving:

- **Fat Content**: 21.2 g
- **Total Net Carbs**: 12 g
- **Protein**: 31.3 g
- **Calories**: 357

List of Ingredients:

- Sausage (1 lb.)
- Diced onion (.5 of 1 small)
- Garlic powder (1 tsp.)
- Diced red bell pepper (1)
- Sautéed mushrooms (3 oz.)
- Tomato paste (1 tbsp.)
- Mozzarella cheese (3 oz.)
- Sliced ham (2 oz.)
- Onion powder (1 tsp.)
- Italian seasoning (1 tsp.)

Preparation Technique:

1. Set the oven at 350° Fahrenheit.
2. Break the sausage apart and smash onto the sides and bottom of the pan.

3. Once loaded, arrange the pan in the heated oven.
4. Bake for 10 to 15 minutes. Transfer it to a platter when done.
5. Combine the garlic powder, tomato paste, Italian seasoning, onion powder, and garlic powder. Sprinkle over the crust.
6. To prepare, just layer with the ham, onions, mushrooms, and red pepper. Give it a sprinkle of mozzarella cheese.
7. Cook for 12 to 15 minutes until golden and the cheese is melted.

Thin Crust White Pizza

Yields Provided: 4 Servings

Macro Counts For Each Serving:

- **Fat Content**: 28.9 g
- **Total Net Carbs**: 4.6 g
- **Protein**: 20 g
- **Calories**: 352

List of Ingredients - The Crust:

- Unflavored egg white protein powder (.25 cup)
- Almond flour (.5 cup)
- Grated parmesan cheese (.5 cup)
- Sea salt/pink Himalayan (.25 tsp.)
- Large egg (1)

List of Ingredients - The Topping:

- Cream cheese (2 tbsp.)
- Onion or garlic powder (1 tsp.)
- Hard-goat cheese/your choice (.5 cup)
- Heavy whipping cream (1 tbsp.)
- Crumbled feta cheese (.33 cup)
- Small red onion (1)
- Seedless Kalamata olives (.25 cup)
- Olive oil (1 tbsp.)

Preparation Technique

1. Set the temperature of the oven to 400° Fahrenheit.
2. Line an iron skillet or a cookie sheet with a piece of parchment paper.
3. Whisk each of the dry fixings in a mixing dish. Blend in the egg - mixing by hand. Empty the batter into the baking pan, spreading evenly. Bake for 10 to 15 min.
4. Prepare the white sauce by mixing the onion/garlic powder, cream cheese, and cream until well combined.
5. Remove the skin from the onion and slice. Grate the hard cheese and crumble the feta. You can also chop the olives.
6. Remove the crust when browned and add the white sauce, both types of cheeses, olives, and onion.
7. Arrange the pan in the oven for another 10 minutes. Remove and slice into quarters. Top with some lettuce leaves with a drizzle of olive oil.

Zucchini Pizza Crust

Yields Provided: 8 Servings

Macro Counts For Each Serving:

- **Fat Content:** 4 g
- **Total Net Carbs:** 2 g
- **Protein:** 6 g
- **Calories:** 83

List of Ingredients:

- Zucchini (8 oz. /about 2 cups grated coarsely, packed loosely into the measuring cup)
- Eggs (3 large)
- Shredded mozzarella cheese - use either pre-shredded or hard mozzarella from a block, not soft fresh (1 cup)
- Coconut flour (.25 cup)
- Sea salt (.5 tsp. + a little more for sprinkling in step 2)
- _Also Needed_: 12 or 14-inch non-stick pizza pan

Preparation Technique:

1. Set the oven to 350° Fahrenheit. Grease the pan. Use parchment paper as an alternative.
2. Spread out the grated zucchini onto the pan in a thin layer. Sprinkle very lightly with a little sea salt. Bake for

about 10-15 minutes, until the zucchini is semi-soft and fairly dry.

3. Meanwhile, combine the eggs, mozzarella, coconut flour and 1/2 tsp sea salt in a large bowl.

4. When the zucchini is done, pat dry as well as possible with paper towels. Mix into the bowl.

5. Lightly wipe down the pizza pan to get rid of any stuck-on zucchini. Cover with parchment paper or grease the pan.

6. Spread the zucchini pizza dough into a thin circle, about 11-12-inch in diameter.

7. Bake for 20-30 minutes, until there are brown spots on the top.

8. Remove the zucchini pizza crust from the oven. Increase the oven temperature to 400° Fahrenheit.

9. Let the crust rest for 10 minutes at room temperature, then top with thick sauce and toppings.

10. Return the zucchini crust pizza to the oven for about 10 minutes, until the cheese on top melts. If desired, place under broiler for 2-3 minutes to brown the cheese.

Chapter 8: Sweets & Snacks

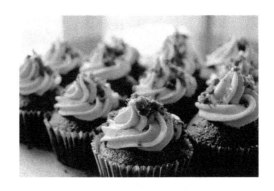

Grain-Free Coffee Walnut Bars

Yields Provided: 14 Servings

Macro Counts For Each Serving:

- **Fat Content**: 11 g
- **Total Net Carbs**: 1.9 g
- **Protein**: 4 g
- **Calories**: 160

List of Ingredients:

- Melted butter (0.5 of 1 stick)
- Granulated sweetener of choice (5 tbsp. more as desired)
- Vanilla (2 tsp.)
- Strong coffee (.5 cup)

- Salt (1 pinch)
- Baking powder (1 tsp.)
- Coconut flour (.66 cup)
- Medium eggs (8)
- Chopped walnuts (.5 cup)

Preparation Technique:

1. Prepare a baking dish with parchment paper. Set the oven at 350° Fahrenheit.
2. Melt and mix the butter, sweetener, and vanilla.
3. Pour in the coffee, baking powder, salt, and flour. Mix gently.
4. Slowly add the eggs and mix.
5. Fold in the chopped walnuts.
6. Pour into a baking dish lined with baking parchment paper. Cook for 15 minutes.
7. Cool, slice into bars. Serve with whipped sweetened cream and a few walnuts.

Hazelnut & Cranberry Crisps

Yields Provided: 18 Servings (64 approx.)

Macro Counts For Each Serving:

- **Fat Content**: 12.87 g
- **Total Net Carbs**: 2.8 g
- **Protein**: 5.96 g
- **Calories**: 115

List of Ingredients:

- Large organic eggs (2)
- Unsweetened dried cranberries (.5 cup)
- Roasted hazelnuts (.5 cup)
- Pumpkin seeds (.33 cup)
- Almond flour (3 cups)
- Erythritol sweetener - brown sugar version is best (.25 cup)
- Baking soda (2 tsp.)
- Salt (.5 tsp.)
- Water (.5 - .75 cup)
- Apple cider vinegar (1 tbsp.)
- Also Needed: 4 mini loaf pans

Preparation Technique:

1. Warm up the oven to 350° Fahrenheit.

2. Prepare the pans with a spritz of oil.

3. Finely chop the hazelnuts, pumpkin seeds, and cranberries. Combine with the sweetener, flour, salt, and baking soda.

4. Stir in the eggs with .5 cup of the water and the vinegar. It should be thick, but it should scoop into the prepared pans. You can add more water if needed (1 tbsp. at a time).

5. Portion into the pans and bake for 30-35 minutes.

6. They should be firm when touched. Let the bread cool in the pan. Place in the freezer for at least one hour – maybe two hours - before slicing.

7. Warm them up. Heat the oven to 250° Fahrenheit.

8. Slice the bread (no more than .25-inch thick).

9. Bake until browned (20-30 min.), and firm to touch. Let the crisps stay in the oven to cool.

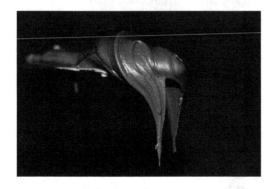

Yields Provided: 32 tablespoons

Macro Counts For Each Serving:

- **Fat Content**: 6 g
- **Total Net Carbs**: 1 g
- **Protein**: 2 g
- **Calories**: 67

List of Ingredients:

- Hazelnuts - preferably raw (2 cups)
- Powdered erythritol (.66 cup or to taste)
- Cocoa powder (unsweetened (.25 cup)
- Avocado oil (or any mild liquid oil of choice (1-2 tbsp.)
- Vanilla extract (1 tsp.)

Preparation Technique:

1. Set the oven to 400° Fahrenheit.

2. Line a sheet with baker paper.

3. Arrange the hazelnuts in a single layer on the baking sheet. Roast for 7 to 10 minutes, until they are browned.

4. Scoop the hazelnuts into a large container with a lid. Shake vigorously to remove the loose skins. Repeat the process as needed, setting aside hazelnuts that already have their skins removed, until most of the skins are off.

5. Place the skinned hazelnuts into a high-power blender, like the Blendtec 625. Process for one to three minutes.

6. Add the cocoa powder, avocado oil (start with 1 tbsp.), cocoa powder, powdered erythritol, and vanilla extract. Process one to two minutes, until the spread is smooth.

7. Add small portions of avocado oil, a teaspoon at a time, if it's too thick. Process again until you reach the desired consistency.

Keto Chocolate Pecan Fudge

Yields Provided: 16 Servings

Macro Counts For Each Serving:

- **Fat Content**: 12 g
- **Total Net Carbs**: 1 g
- **Protein**: 1 g
- **Calories**: 112

List of Ingredients:

- Butter (.25 cup)
- Coconut oil (.25 cup)
- Cream cheese (1 cup)
- Pecans (.5 cup)
- Vanilla extract (1 tbsp.)
- Cocoa powder (.125 cup)
- Powdered sweetener (3 tbsp.)

Preparation Technique:

1. Chop the pecans using a food processor or sharp knife.
2. Combine the softened butter, cream cheese, and coconut oil using a hand mixer.
3. Add the pecans, cocoa powder, vanilla extract, and sweetener. Mix well.

4. Scoop the batter into a baking pan. Cool for at least 2 hours or until set.
5. Using a knife, cut the keto fudge into little squares.
6. Store them in the fridge.

2-Minute Peanut Butter Mini Cake

Yields Provided: 2 Servings

Macro Counts For Each Serving:

- **Fat Content**: 16 g
- **Total Net Carbs**: 6 g
- **Protein**: 7 g
- **Calories**: 215

List of Ingredients - The Batter:

- Melted butter or coconut oil (1.5 tbsp.)
- Unsweetened coconut milk/Heavy cream (1 tbsp.)
- Vanilla extract (.25 tsp.)
- Large egg (1)
- Almond or Peanut butter (1.5 tbsp.)
- Baking soda (.25 tsp.)
- Coconut flour - divided (1 tbsp. & 1 tsp.)
- Swerve/another favorite (2 tbsp.)
- Apple cider vinegar (.5 tsp.)
- *Optional*: Sugar-free chocolate chips (1 tbsp.)

List of Ingredients - Frosting Ingredients:

- Almond/peanut butter (2.5 tbsp.)
- Vanilla extract (.125 tsp.)
- Cocoa powder (1.5 tsp.)

- Swerve (1 tbsp.)
- *Optional:* Add for thinning - Coconut oil (.5 tsp.)
- Also Needed: 7-8-inch (16-32 oz. glass bowl)

Preparation Technique:

1. Prepare the batter. Add 1.5 tbsp. melted butter/oil into the chosen bowl.
2. Add heavy cream, one large egg, vanilla extract, and almond butter. Whisk fully; and mix in the coconut flour, and sweetener of choice.
3. Whisk in the baking soda, vinegar, and chocolate chips.
4. Microwave on high for 1.5 min. Then let it cool.
5. Prepare the frosting.
6. Loosen the cake. Dump the container over onto a plate.
7. Cut in half. Frost both layers and serve.

Pancakes

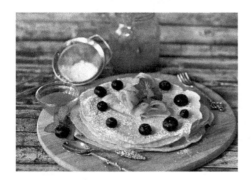

Sweet Pancakes

Yields Provided: 4 Servings

Macro Counts For Each Serving:

- **Fat Content**: 33 g
- **Total Net Carbs**: 7 g
- **Protein**: 4 g
- **Calories**: 345

List of Ingredients:

- Unchilled butter (2 oz.)
- Pecans or walnuts (1 oz.)
- Coconut flour (4 tbsp.)
- Ground cinnamon (.5 tsp.)

- Vanilla extract (.25 tsp.)
- Tart/sour apple (1)

List of Ingredients - For Serving:
- Heavy whipping cream (.75 cup)
- Vanilla extract (.5 tsp.)

Preparation Technique:
1. Program the oven to 350° Fahrenheit. Mix coconut flour, cinnamon, softened butter, chopped nuts, and vanilla into a crumbly dough.
2. Cut off both ends and cut the middle part in four slices.
3. Place the slices in a greased baking dish and add dough crumbs on top. Bake until the crumbs turn golden brown (15 min.).
4. Add vanilla and whipping cream and vanilla into a mixing container and whip until soft peaks form.
5. Cool for 30 min and serve with whipped cream.

Walnut Pancakes

Yields Provided: 3 Servings

Macro Counts For Each Serving:

- **Fat Content**: 18 g
- **Total Net Carbs**: 8 g
- **Protein**: 6 g
- **Calories**: 227

List of Ingredients:

- Ground walnuts (.66 cup)
- Coconut flour (1.5 tbsp.)
- Baking powder (.5 tsp.)
- Pure maple syrup (1 tbsp.)
- Egg (1)
- Almond milk (2 tbsp.)
- Vanilla extract (.5 tsp.)

Preparation Technique:

1. Spray a pan with oil spray, and warm up on the stovetop using the medium heat temperature setting.
2. Combine the dry fixings, and add the egg, vanilla, and syrup.

3. Pour in milk and mix until combined. Portion into three even circles.
4. Cook (the lid off) for six minutes.
5. Flip and cook another three to four minutes until.
6. Turn the pan off and cover. Let it sit for two minutes to finish cooking.

Conclusion

I hope you have thoroughly enjoyed each chapter of *Keto Bread*. I also hope it was informative and provided you with all of the tools you need to achieve your goals whatever they may be. The next step is to decide which delicious treat you want to make first. Head to the store for the fixings and you are ready to start.

If you are using the keto plan for weight loss, you may not see any results at first.

There could be days or weeks where you don't see the changes, but slow is the best method. You are altering your lifestyle and breaking old habits. You need to remain patient because there aren't any quick fixes to weight loss. As with any new challenge, the initial phase of a long-term trial is difficult.

You have to realize it takes time for your body to accommodate the ketogenic diet plan. It can take anywhere from two to four weeks or more. For some, it can take as much as six to eight weeks. It takes time because you cannot instantly switch over to using fat as a fuel source. It takes time for your body to adjust to the changes. You may be experiencing low energy, withdrawal-type symptoms, fatigue, or headaches, but they will pass.

Some recipes might not be 100% keto-friendly. You can also adjust the ingredients to your own discretion. Remember this Formula: Total Carbs minus (-) Fiber = Net Carbs. This is the logic used for each of the recipes included in this cookbook and guidelines.

Walk away with the knowledge learned and prepare a feast using your delicious new bread recipes and other delicious options. Be the envy of the neighborhood when you provide a feast at the next neighborhood gathering. Show off your skills and be proud. You can also boast of how much better you feel using the ketogenic diet plan.

After you have started losing your weight, it's essential to have a bit of fun. However, you should be sure it is not a food-related treat unless it's keto-friendly. Buy a new outfit to show off your weight loss. Take the family for an evening on-the-town. You deserve it.

Finally, if you found this book useful in any way, a review on Amazon is always appreciated!

CPSIA information can be obtained
at www.ICGtesting.com
Printed in the USA
LVHW080806100221
678883LV00002B/67